TASTY

ANTI-INFLAMMATORY

RECIPES 2021

EASY RECIPES TO HEAL THE IMMUNE SYSTEM

DIANA SMITH

Table of Contents

Oatmeal Pancakes *Servings: 1*

Cooking Time: 10 Minutes

Ingredients:

Egg – 1

Rolled oats, ground – 0.5 cup

Almond milk – 2 tablespoons

Baking soda – 0.125 teaspoon

Baking powder – 0.125 teaspoon

Vanilla extract – 1 teaspoon

Date paste – 1 teaspoon

Directions:

1. Warm up your non-stick griddle or skillet over medium while you prepare the pancakes.

2. Place the rolled oats into your blender or food processor and pulse until they grind into a fine flour. Add them to a bowl, whisking them with the baking powder and baking soda.

3. In another kitchen bowl, whisk together the egg with almond milk, date paste, and vanilla extract until combined. Add the sweetened egg/almond milk mixture to the oat flour mixture and fold together just until combined.

4. Grease your skillet and then ladle on your pancake batter leaving a bit of room between each pancake. Allow your pancakes to cook for about two to three minutes, until golden-brown and bubbly.

Carefully, flip over the pancakes and cook the other side for a couple of minutes until it is golden, as well.

5. Remove your pancakes from the stove and serve them with your choice of fruit, yogurt, compote, or Lakanto's monk fruit maple-flavored syrup.

Maple Oatmeal _Servings: 4_

Cooking Time: 20 Minutes

Ingredients:

Maple flavoring, one teaspoon

Cinnamon, one teaspoon

Sunflower seeds, three tablespoons

Pecans, one-half cup chopped

Coconut flakes, unsweetened, one quarter cup Walnuts, one-half cup chopped

Milk, almond or coconut, one half cup

Chia seeds, four tablespoons

Directions:

1. Pulse the sunflower seeds, walnuts, and pecans in a food processor to crumble. Or you can just put the nuts in a sturdy plastic bag, wrap the bag with a towel, lay it on a sturdy surface, and beat the towel with a hammer until the nuts are crumbled. Mix the crushed nuts with the rest of the ingredients and pour them into a large pot.

Simmer this mixture over low heat for thirty minutes. Stir often, so the mix does not stick to the bottom. Serve garnished with fresh fruit or a sprinkle of cinnamon if desired.

Nutrition Info: Calories 374 carbs 3.2 grams protein 9.25 grams fat 34.59 grams

Kiwi Strawberry Smoothie _Servings: 1_

Cooking Time: 0 Minutes

Ingredients:

Kiwi, peeled and chopped, one

Strawberries, fresh or frozen, one-half cup chopped Milk, almond or coconut, one cup

Basil, ground, one teaspoon

Turmeric, one teaspoon

Banana, diced, one

Chia seed powder, one quarter cup

Directions:

1. Drink immediately after all the ingredients have been well mixed.

Nutrition Info: Calories 250 sugar 9.9 grams fat 1-gram grams 34

carbs fiber 4.3 grams

Flaxseed Porridge With Cinnamon _Servings: 4_

Cooking Time: 5 Minutes

Ingredients:

1 tsp cinnamon

1½ tsp stevia

1 tbsp unsalted butter

2 tbsp flaxseed meal

2 tbsp flaxseed oatmeal

½ cup shredded coconut

1 cup heavy cream

2 cups of water

Directions:

1. Take a medium pot, place it over low heat, add all the ingredients in it, stir until mixed and bring the mixture to boil.

2. When the mixture has boiled, remove the pot from heat, stir it well and divide it evenly between four bowls.

3. Let porridge rest for 10 minutes until slightly thicken and then serve.

Nutrition Info: Calories 171, Total Fat 16g, Total Carbs 6g, Protein 2g

Sweet Potato Cranberry Breakfast Bars

Servings: 8

Cooking Time: 40 Minutes

Ingredients:

1 ½ cups sweet potato puree

2 tablespoons coconut oil, melted

2 tablespoons maple syrup

2 eggs, pasture-raised

1 cup almond meal

1/3 cup coconut flour

1 ½ teaspoon baking soda

1 cup fresh cranberry, pitted and chopped

¼ cup water

Directions:

1. Preheat the oven to 3500F.

2. Grease a 9-inch baking pan with coconut oil. Set aside.

3. In a mixing bowl. Combine the sweet potato puree, water, coconut oil, maple syrup, and eggs.

4. In another bowl, sift the almond flour, coconut flour, and baking soda.

5. Gradually add the dry ingredients to the wet ingredients. Use a spatula to fold and mix all ingredients.

6. Pour into the prepared baking pan and press the cranberries on top.

7. Place in the oven and bake for 40 minutes or until a toothpick inserted in the middle comes out clean.

8. Allow to rest or cool before removing from the pan.

Nutrition Info: Calories 98Total Fat 6gSaturated Fat 1gTotal Carbs 9gNet Carbs 8.5gProtein 3gSugar: 7gFiber: 0.5gSodium: 113

mgPotassium 274mg

Pumpkin Spice Baked Oatmeal <u>*Servings: 6*</u>

Cooking Time: 35 Minutes

Ingredients:

Rolled oats – 1.5 cups

Almond milk, unsweetened – 0.75 cup

Egg – 1

Lakanto monk fruit sweetener – 0.5 cup

Pumpkin puree – 1 cup

Vanilla extract – 1 teaspoon

Pecans, chopped – 0.75 cup

Baking powder – 1 teaspoon

Sea salt – 0.5 teaspoon

Pumpkin pie spice – 1.5 teaspoons

Directions:

1. Warm your oven to Fahrenheit 350 degrees and grease an eight-by-eight baking dish.

2. In a bowl, whisk together the rolled oats, almond milk, eggs, and remaining ingredients until the oatmeal batter is fully combined. Pour the pumpkin spiced oatmeal mixture into your greased pan and place it in the center of your oven.

3. Bake your oatmeal until it is golden in color and set, about twenty-five to thirty minutes. Remove the pumpkin spice baked oatmeal from the oven and allow it to cool for five minutes before serving. Enjoy warm alone or with your favorite fruit and yogurt.

Spinach And Tomato Egg Scramble _Servings: 1_

Ingredients:

1 tsp. olive oil

1 tsp. chopped fresh basil

1 medium chopped tomato

¼ c. Swiss cheese

2 eggs

½ tsp. cayenne pepper

½ c. chopped packed spinach

Directions:

1. In a small bowl, whisk well eggs, basil, pepper, and Swiss cheese.

2. Place a medium fry pan on medium fire and heat oil.

3. Stir in tomato and sauté for 3 minutes. Stir in spinach and cook for 2 minutes or until starting to wilt.

4. Pour in beaten eggs and scramble for 2 to 3 minutes or to desired doneness.

5. Enjoy.

<u>Nutrition Info:</u> Calories: 230, Fat:14.3 g, Carbs:8.4 g, Protein:17.9

Tropical Carrot Ginger And Turmeric Smoothie

Servings: 1

Cooking Time: 0 Minutes

Ingredients:

1 blood orange, peeled and seeded

1 large carrot, peeled and chopped

½ cup frozen mango chunks

2/3 cup coconut water

1 tablespoon raw hemp seeds

¾ teaspoon grated ginger

1 ½ teaspoon peeled and grated turmeric

A pinch of cayenne pepper

A pinch of salt

Directions:

1. Place all ingredients in a blender and blend until smooth.

2. Chill before serving.

<u>Nutrition Info:</u> Calories 259Total Fat 6gSaturated Fat 0.9gTotal Carbs 51gNet Carbs 40gProtein 7gSugar: 34gFiber: 11gSodium: 225mgPotassium 1319mg

French Toast With Cinnamon Vanilla

Servings: 4

Ingredients:

½ tsp. cinnamon

3 large eggs

1 tsp. vanilla

8 whole-wheat slices bread

2 tbsps. Low-fat milk

Directions:

1. First, preheat a griddle to 3500F.

2. Combine the vanilla, eggs, milk, and cinnamon in a small bowl and whisk until smooth.

3. Pour into a plate or flat-bottomed dish.

4. Into the egg mixture, dip the bread, flip to coat both sides and put on the hot griddle.

5. Cook for about 2 minutes or until the bottom is lightly browned, then flip and cook the other side as well.

Nutrition Info: Calories: 281.0, Fat:10.8 g, Carbs:37.2 g, Protein:14.5 g, Sugars:10 g, Sodium:390 mg.

Breakfast Avocado Boat *Servings: 2*

Cooking Time: 7 Minutes

Ingredients:

2 avocados, sliced in half and pitted

¼ onion, chopped

2 tomatoes, chopped

1 bell pepper, chopped

2 tablespoons cilantro, chopped

Pepper to taste

4 eggs

Directions:

1. Scoop out the flesh of the avocado and chop.

2. Place in a bowl.

3. Stir in the rest of the ingredients except.

4. Refrigerate for 30 minutes.

5. Crack egg on top of avocado shell.

6. Preheat your air fryer to 350 degrees F.

7. Air fry for 7 minutes.

8. Top with avocado salsa.

Turkey Hash <u>Servings: 4</u>

Cooking Time: 15 Minutes

Ingredients:

1-pound ground turkey

½ teaspoon dried thyme

1 tablespoon coconut oil, melted

½ teaspoon ground cinnamon

For the hash:

1 yellow onion, chopped

1 tablespoon coconut oil, melted

1 zucchini, chopped

½ cup shredded carrots

2 cups butternut squash, cubed

1 apple, cored, peeled and cubed

2 cups baby spinach

1 teaspoon ground ginger

1 teaspoon ground cinnamon

½ teaspoon garlic powder

½ teaspoon turmeric powder

½ teaspoon dried thyme

Directions:

1. Heat up a pan with 1 tablespoon coconut oil over medium-high heat. Add the turkey, ½ teaspoon thyme and ½ teaspoon ground cinnamon. Mix and cook for 5 minutes then transfer to a bowl. Heat up the pan again with 1 tablespoon coconut oil over medium-high heat. Add the onion, stir and cook for 2 minutes. Add the zucchini, the carrots, squash, apple, ginger, 1 teaspoon cinnamon, ½

teaspoon thyme, turmeric and garlic powder. Stir and cook for 3-4

minutes. Return the meat to the pan, also add the baby spinach. Mix together and cook for 1-2 minutes more then divide everything between plates and serve for breakfast.

2. Enjoy!

Nutrition Info: calories 212, fat 4, fiber 6, carbs 8, protein 7

Steel Cut Oats With Kefir And Berries

Servings: 4

Cooking Time: 30 Minutes

Ingredients:

For the oats:

1 cup steel-cut oats

3 cups of water

pinch of salt

For topping Optional:

fresh or frozen fruit/berries

a handful of sliced almonds, hemp seeds, pepitas, or other nuts/seeds

unsweetened kefir, homemade/store-bought

a drizzle of maple syrup, sprinkling of coconut sugar, a few drops of stevia, or any other sweetener you like, to taste Directions:

1. Add/place the oats in a small saucepan and over medium-high heat. Make the pan toast, often stir or shake, for 2-3 minutes.

2. Adding the water and bring to a boil. Reduce heat to a cooker and let it cook for about 25 minutes, or until the oats are soft enough to satisfy you. Serve with berries, nuts/seeds, a splash of kefir, and any sweetener you like, to taste. Dig in!

<u>Nutrition Info:</u> Calories 150 Carbs: 27g Fat: 3g Protein: 4g

Fantastic Spaghetti Squash With Cheese And Basil Pesto

Servings: 2

Cooking Time: 35 Minutes

Ingredients:

1 cup cooked spaghetti squash, drained

Salt and freshly cracked black pepper, to taste ½ tbsp olive oil

¼ cup ricotta cheese, unsweetened

2oz fresh mozzarella cheese, cubed

1/8 cup basil pesto

Directions:

1. Switch on the oven, then set its temperature to 375 °F and let it preheat.

2. Meanwhile, take a medium bowl, add spaghetti squash in it and then season with salt and black pepper.

3. Take a casserole dish, grease it with oil, add squash mixture in it, top it with ricotta cheese and mozzarella cheese and bake for 10

minutes until cooked.

4. When done, remove the casserole dish from the oven, drizzle pesto on top and serve immediately.

<u>Nutrition Info:</u> Calories 169, Total Fat 11.3g, Total Carbs 6.2g, Protein 11.9g, Sugar 0.1g, Sodium 217mg

Hearty Orange Peach Smoothie <u>*Servings: 2*</u>

Ingredients:

2 c. chopped peaches

2 tbsps. Unsweetened yogurt

Juice of 2 oranges

Directions:

1. Start by removing the seeds and peel from the peaches. Chop and leave some chunks of peach for topping.

2. Place the chopped peach, orange juice and yogurt in a blender and run until smooth.

3. You may add some water to thin the smoothie if you want.

4. Pour into glass cups and enjoy!

<u>Nutrition Info:</u> Calories: 170, Fat:4.5 g, Carbs:28 g, Protein:7 g, Sugars:23 g, Sodium:101 mg

Banana Almond Butter Muffins <u>Servings: 6</u>

Cooking Time: 30 Minutes

Ingredients:

Oat flour – 1 cup

Sea salt – 0.25 teaspoon

Cinnamon, ground – 0.5 teaspoon

Baking powder – 1 teaspoon

Almond butter – 0.75 cup

Banana, mashed – 1 cup

Almond milk, unsweetened – 0.5 tablespoon

Vanilla extract – 2 teaspoons

Eggs – 2

Lakanto monk fruit sweetener – 0.25 cup

Directions:

1. Warm your oven to Fahrenheit 350 degrees and line a muffin tin with paper liners or grease it if you would rather.

2. In a kitchen bowl, whisk together your mashed banana with the almond butter, unsweetened almond milk, eggs, vanilla extract, and monk fruit sweetener. In a separate kitchen mixing dish, combine together the oat flour, spices, and baking powder. Once the flour mixture is fully combined, pour it into the bowl with the mashed banana and fold both the almond butter/banana mixture and the oat flour mixtures together just until combined.

3. Divide the muffin batter between the twelve paper liners, filling each muffin cavity about three-quarters of the way full. Place the banana almond butter muffins tin in the middle of your hot oven and allow them to cook until set and cooked through. They are done once a toothpick is pricked inside the center and removed cleanly.

This should take about twenty to twenty-five minutes.

4. Allow the banana almond butter muffins to cool before serving, and then enjoy.

Breakfast Porridge Servings: 1

Cooking Time: 0 Minutes;

Ingredients:

6 tablespoons organic cottage cheese

3 tablespoons flaxseed

3 tablespoons flax oil

2 tablespoons organic raw almond butter

1 tablespoon organic coconut meat

1 tablespoon raw honey

¼ cup water

Directions:

1. Combine all ingredients in a bowl. Mix until well combined.

2. Place in a bowl and chill before serving.

Nutrition Info: Calories 632Total Fat 49gSaturated Fat 5gTotal Carbs 32gNet Carbs 26gProtein 23gSugar: 22g Fiber: 6gSodium: 265mg Potassium 533mg

Banana Bread Overnight Oats _Servings: 3_

Cooking Time: 0 Minutes

Ingredients:

¼-cup plain Greek yogurt

¼-tsp flaked sea salt

1½-cups nonfat milk

1-cup old-fashioned rolled oats

1-Tbsp chia seeds

2-pcs medium bananas, very ripe and mashed

2-Tbsps coconut flakes, unsweetened and toasted 2-Tbsps honey

2-tsp vanilla extract

Toppings for serving: roasted pecans, pomegranate seeds, honey, fig halves, and banana slices

Directions:

1. Stir in all of the ingredients, excluding the toppings, in a mixing bowl. Mix well until thoroughly combined. Divide the mixture equally between two serving bowls.

2. Cover and refrigerate overnight or for 6 hours.

3. To serve, stir, and put on the toppings.

Nutrition Info: Calories 684 Fat: 22.8g Protein: 34.2g Sodium: 374mg Total Carbs: 99.6g Dietary Fiber: 14.1g

Choco Chia Banana Bowl _Servings: 3_

Cooking Time: 0 Minutes

Ingredients:

½-cup chia seeds

1 large banana, very ripe

½-tsp pure vanilla extract

2-cups almond milk, unsweetened

1-Tbsp cacao powder

2-Tbsps raw honey or maple syrup

2-Tbsps cacao nibs for mixing in

2-Tbsps chocolate chips for mixing in

1 large banana, sliced for mixing in

Directions:

1. Combine the chia seeds and banana in a mixing bowl. By using a fork, mash the banana and mix well until thoroughly combined. Pour in the vanilla and almond milk. Whisk until no more lumps appear.

2. Pour half of the mix in a glass container, and cover it. Add the cacao and syrup to the remaining half mixture in the bowl. Mix well until fully incorporated. Pour this mixture in another glass container, and cover it. Chill for at least 4 hours.

3. To serve, layer the chilled chia puddings equally in three serving bowls. Alternate the layers with the ingredients for mixing-in.

<u>Nutrition Info:</u> Calories 293 Fat: 9.7g Protein: 14.6g Sodium: 35mg Total Carbs: 43.1g

Anti-inflammatory Cherry Spinach Smoothie

Servings: 1

Cooking Time: 0 Minutes

Ingredients:

1 cup plain kefir

1 cup frozen cherries, pitted

½ cup baby spinach leaves

¼ cup mashed ripe avocado

1 tablespoon almond butter

1-piece peeled ginger (1/2 inch)

1 teaspoon chia seeds

Directions:

1. Place all ingredients in a blender.

2. Pulse until smooth.

3. Allow to chill in the fridge before serving.

<u>Nutrition Info:</u> Calories 410Total Fat 20gSaturated Fat 4gTotal Carbs 47gNet Carbs 37gProtein 17gSugar: 33gFiber: 10gSodium: 169mgPotassium 1163mg

Spicy Shakshuka _Servings: 4_

Cooking Time: 37 Minutes

Ingredients:

2-Tbsps extra-virgin olive oil

1-bulb onion, minced

1 jalapeño, seeded and minced

2-cloves garlic, minced

1-lb spinach

Salt and freshly ground black pepper

¾-tsp coriander

1-tsp dried cumin

2-Tbsps harissa paste

½-cup vegetable broth

8-pcs large eggs

Red pepper flakes, for serving

Cilantro, chopped for serving

Parsley, chopped for serving

Directions:

1. Preheat your oven to 350°F.

2. Heat the oil in an oven-safe skillet placed over medium heat. Stir in the onion and sauté for 5 minutes.

3. Add the jalapeño and garlic, and sauté for a minute, or until fragrant. Add in the spinach, and cook for 5 minutes, or until the leaves entirely wilt.

4. Season the mixture with salt and pepper, coriander, cumin, and harissa. Cook further for 1 minute.

5. Transfer the mixture to your food processor—puree to a thick consistency. Pour in the broth and puree further until achieving a smooth texture.

6. Clean and grease the same skillet with nonstick cooking spray.

Pour the pureed mixture. By using a wooden spoon, form eight circular wells.

7. Crack each egg gently into the wells. Put the skillet in the oven—

Bake for 25 minutes, or poaching the eggs until fully set.

8. To serve, sprinkle the shakshuka with red pepper flakes, cilantro, and parsley to taste.

<u>Nutrition Info:</u> Calories 251 Fat: 8.3g Protein: 12.5g Sodium: 165mg Total Carbs: 33.6g

5-minute Golden Milk _Servings: 1_

Cooking Time: 4 Minutes

Ingredients:

1 1/2 cups light coconut milk

1 1/2 cups unsweetened almond milk

1 1/2 tsp ground turmeric

1/4 tsp ground ginger

1 whole cinnamon stick

1 Tbsp coconut oil

1 pinch ground black pepper

Sweetener of choice (i.e., coconut sugar, maple syrup, or stevia to taste)

Directions:

1. Add coconut milk, ground turmeric, almond milk, ground ginger, cinnamon stick, coconut oil, black pepper, and preferred sweetener to a small casserole.

2. Whisk to mix over medium heat and warm up. Heat to the touch until hot but do not boil-about 4 minutes-whisking regularly.

3. Turn off heat and taste to make flavor change. For strong spice + flavor, add more sweetener to taste, or more turmeric or ginger.

4. Serve straight away, break between two glasses, and leave the cinnamon stick behind. Best when fresh, although the leftovers can be kept 2-3 days in the refrigerator. Reheat up to temperature on the stovetop or microwave.

Nutrition Info: Calories 205 Fat: 19.5g Sodium: 161mg Carbohydrates: 8.9g Fiber: 1.1g Protein: 3.2g

Breakfast Oatmeal _Servings: 1_

Cooking Time: 8 Minutes

Ingredients:

2/3 cup coconut milk

1 egg white, pasture-raised

½ cup gluten-free quick-cooking oats

½ teaspoon turmeric powder

½ teaspoon cinnamon

¼ teaspoon ginger

Directions:

1. Place the non-dairy milk in a saucepan and heat over medium flame.

2. Stir in the egg white and continue whisking until the mixture becomes smooth.

3. Add in the rest of the ingredients and cook for another 3 minutes.

Nutrition Info: Calories 395Total Fat 34gSaturated Fat 7gTotal Carbs 19gNet Carbs 16gProtein 10gSugar: 2gFiber: 3gSodium: 76mgPotassium 459mg

No-bake Turmeric Protein Donuts _Servings: 8_

Cooking Time: 0 Minutes

Ingredients:

1 ½ cups raw cashews

½ cup medjool dates, pitted

1 tablespoon vanilla protein powder

½ cup shredded coconut

2 tablespoons maple syrup

¼ teaspoon vanilla extract

1 teaspoon turmeric powder

¼ cup dark chocolate

Directions:

1. Combine all ingredients except for the chocolate in a food processor.

2. Pulse until smooth.

3. Roll batter into 8 balls and press into a silicone donut mold.

4. Place in the freezer for 30 minutes to set.

5. Meanwhile, make the chocolate topping by melting the chocolate in a double boiler.

6. Once the donuts have set, remove the donuts from the mold and drizzle with chocolate.

Nutrition Info: Calories 320Total Fat 26gSaturated Fat 5gTotal Carbs 20gNet Carbs 18gProtein 7gSugar: 9gFiber: 2gSodium: 163

mgPotassium 297mg

Cheddar & Kale Frittata *Servings: 6*

Ingredients:

1/3 c. sliced scallions

¼ tsp. pepper

1 diced red pepper

¾ c. non-fat milk

1 c. shredded sharp low-fat cheddar cheese

1 tsp. olive oil

5 oz. baby kale and spinach

12 eggs

Directions:

1. Preheat oven to 375 0F.

2. With olive oil, grease a glass casserole dish.

3. In a bowl, whisk well all ingredients except for cheese.

4. Pour egg mixture in prepared dish and bake for 35 minutes.

5. Remove from oven and sprinkle cheese on top and broil for 5 minutes.

6. Remove from oven and let it sit for 10 minutes.

7. Cut up and enjoy.

Nutrition Info: Calories: 198, Fat:11.0 g, Carbs:5.7 g, Protein:18.7 g, Sugars:1 g, Sodium:209 mg.

Mediterranean Frittata _Servings: 6_

Cooking Time: 20 Minutes

Ingredients:

Eggs, six

Feta cheese, crumbled, one quarter cup

Black pepper, one quarter teaspoon

Oil, spray, or olive

Oregano, one teaspoon

Milk, almond or coconut, one quarter cup

Sea salt, one teaspoon

Black olives, chopped, one quarter cup

Green olives, chopped, one quarter cup

Tomatoes, diced, one quarter cup

Directions:

1. Heat oven to 400. Oil one eight by eight-inch baking dish.

Combine the milk into the eggs, and then add other ingredients. Pour all of this mixture into the baking dish and bake for twenty minutes.

Nutrition Info: Calories 107 sugars 2 grams fat 7 grams carb 3

grams protein 7 grams

Buckwheat Cinnamon And Ginger Granola

<u>Servings: 5</u>

Cooking Time: 40 Minutes

Ingredients:

¼ cup Chia seeds

½ Cup Coconut Flakes

1 ½ Cup mixed Raw nuts

2 cups of gluten-free oats

1 cup of buckwheat groats

2 tbsp nut butter

4 tbsp of coconut oil

1 cup of sunflower seeds

½ cup of pumpkin seeds

1 ½ - 2 inches piece of ginger

1 tsp Ground Cinnamon

1/3 cup of Rice Malt Syrup

4 tbsp of raw cacao powder – Optional

Directions:

1. Preheat the oven up to 180C

2. Blitz the nuts in your food processor and quickly blitz to chop roughly. Put the chopped nuts in a bowl and add all the other dry ingredients that combine well–oats, coconut, cinnamon, buckwheat, seeds, and salt in a low heat saucepan, melt the coconut oil gently.

3. Add the cacao powder (if used) to the wet mixture and blend. Put the wet batter over the dry mix, then mix well to make sure that everything is coated. Move the mixture to a wide baking tray lined with grease-proof paper or coconut oil greased. Be sure to uniformly distribute the mixture for 35-40 minutes, turning the mixture halfway through. Bake until the granola is fresh and golden!

4. Serve with your favorite nut milk, coconut yogurt scoop, fresh fruit, and superfoods–goji berries, flax seeds, bee pollen, whatever you like! Mix it up every single day.

Nutrition Info: Calories 220 Carbs: 38g Fat: 5g Protein: 7g

Cilantro Pancakes _Servings: 6_

Cooking Time: 6-8 Minutes

Ingredients:

½ cup tapioca flour

½ cup almond flour

½ teaspoon chili powder

¼ teaspoon ground turmeric

Salt and freshly ground black pepper, to taste 1 cup full- Fat coconut milk

½ of red onion, chopped

1 (½-inch) fresh ginger piece, grated finely 1 Serrano pepper, minced

½ cup fresh cilantro, chopped

Oil, as required

Directions:

1. In a big bowl, mix together flours and spices.

2. Add coconut milk and mix till well combined.

3. Fold within the onion, ginger, Serrano pepper and cilantro.

4. Lightly, grease a sizable nonstick skillet with oil and warmth on medium-low heat.

5. Add about ¼ cup of mixture and tilt the pan to spread it evenly inside the skillet.

6. Cook for around 3-4 minutes from either side.

7. Repeat with all the remaining mixture.

8. Serve along with your desired topping.

Nutrition Info: Calories: 331, Fat: 10g, Carbohydrates: 37g, Fiber: 6g, Protein: 28g

Raspberry Grapefruit Smoothie _Servings: 1_

Cooking Time: 0 Minutes

Ingredients:

Juice from 1 grapefruit, freshly squeezed

1 banana, peeled and sliced

1 cup raspberries

Directions:

1. Place all ingredients in a blender and pulse until smooth.

2. Chill before serving.

Nutrition Info: Calories 381Total Fat 0.8gSaturated Fat 0.1gTotal Carbs 96gNet Carbs 85gProtein 4gSugar: 61gFiber: 11gSodium: 11mgPotassium 848mg

Peanut Butter Granola Servings: 8

Cooking Time: 25 Minutes

Ingredients:

Rolled oats – 2 cups

Cinnamon – 0.5 teaspoon

Peanut butter, natural with salt – 0.5 cup

Date paste – 1.5 tablespoons

Lily's dark chocolate chips – 0.5 cup

Directions:

1. Warm the oven to Fahrenheit 300 degrees and line a baking sheet with kitchen parchment or a silicone kitchen mat.

2. In a bowl, whisk together the date paste, cinnamon, and peanut butter to combine, and then add in the oats, tossing until the oats are fully coated. Spread this sweetened and spiced mixture evenly over the baking sheet in a thin layer.

3. Place the peanut butter granola in the oven and bake for twenty minutes, giving it a good stir halfway through the cooking time to prevent uneven cooking and burning.

4. Remove the granola from the oven and allow it to cool to room temperature before tossing in the chocolate chips. Transfer the peanut butter granola to an airtight container to store until use.

Turmeric Oven Scrambled Eggs Servings: 6

Cooking Time: 15 Minutes

Ingredients:

8 to 10 large eggs, pasture-raised

½ cup unsweetened almond or coconut milk

½ teaspoon turmeric powder

1 teaspoon chopped cilantro

¼ teaspoon black pepper

A pinch of salt

Directions:

1. Preheat the oven to 3500F.

2. Grease a casserole or heat-proof baking dish.

3. In a bowl, whisk the egg, milk, turmeric powder, black pepper and salt.

4. Pour in the egg mixture into the baking dish.

5. Place in the oven and bake for 15 minutes or until the eggs have set.

6. Remove from the oven and garnish with chopped cilantro on top.

Nutrition Info: Calories 203Total Fat 16gSaturated Fat 4gTotal Carbs 5gNet Carbs 4gProtein 10gSugar: 4gFiber: 1gSodium: 303

mgPotassium 321mg

Chia And Oat Breakfast Bran _Servings: 2_

Ingredients:

85 g chopped roasted almonds

340 g coconut milk

30 g cane sugar

2½ g orange zest

30 g flax seed mix

170 g rolled oats

340 g blueberries

30 g chia seeds

2½ g cinnamon

Directions:

1. Add all your wet ingredients together and mix the sugar and milk in with the orange zest.

2. Stir in the cinnamon and mix well. Once you are sure the sugar isn't lumpy add in the rolled oats, flax seeds, and chia and then let it sit for a minute.

3. Grab two bowls or mason jars and pour the mixture in. Top with the roasted almonds, and store in the fridge.

4. Pull it out in the morning and dig in!

<u>Nutrition Info:</u> Calories: 353, Fat:8 g, Carbs:55 g, Protein:15 g, Sugars:9.9 g, Sodium:96 mg

Rhubarb, Apple Plus Ginger Muffin Recipe

Servings: 8

Cooking Time: 30 Minutes

Ingredients:

1/2 teaspoon ground cinnamon

1/2 teaspoon ground ginger

pinch sea salt

1/2 cup almond meal (ground almonds)

1/4 cup unrefined raw sugar

2 tbsp finely chopped crystallized ginger

1 tbs ground linseed meal

1/2 cup buckwheat flour

1/4 cup fine brown rice flour

1/4 cup (60ml) olive oil

1 large free-range egg

1 teaspoon vanilla extract

2 tablespoons organic corn flour or true arrowroot 2 teaspoons gluten-free baking powder

1 cup finely sliced rhubarb

1 small apple, peeled and finely diced

95ml (1/3 cup + 1 tbsp) rice or almond milk <u>Directions:</u>

1. Pre-heat the oven to 180C/350C. Grease or line 8 1/3 cup (80ml) cup muffin tins with a paper case cap.

2. In a medium bowl, put the almond meal, ginger, sugar, and linseed. Sieve over baking powder, flours, and spices and then mix evenly. In the flour mixture, whisk in rhubarb and apple to coat.

3. Whisk the milk, sugar, egg, and vanilla in another smaller bowl before pouring into the dry mixture and stirring until combined.

4. Divide the batter evenly between tins/paper cases and bake for 20 minutes -25 minutes or until it rises, golden around the edges.

5. Remove, then set aside for 5 minutes before transferring onto a wire rack to cool off further.

6. Eat warm or at room temperature.

<u>Nutrition Info:</u> Calories 38 Carbs: 9g Fat: 0g Protein: 0g

Breakfast Grains And Fruits *Servings: 6*

Ingredients:

1 c. raisins

¾ c. quick cooking brown rice

1 granny smith apple

1 orange

8 oz. low fat vanilla yogurt

3 c. water

¾ c. bulgur

1 red delicious apple

Directions:

1. On high fire, place a large pot and bring water to a boil.

2. Add bulgur and rice. Lower fire to a simmer and cook for ten minutes while covered.

3. Turn off fire, set aside for 2 minutes while covered.

4. In a baking sheet, transfer and evenly spread grains to cool.

5. Meanwhile, peel oranges and cut into sections. Chop and core apples.

6. Once grains are cool, transfer to a large serving bowl along with fruits.

7. Add yogurt and mix well to coat.

8. Serve and enjoy.

Nutrition Info: Calories: 121, Fat:1 g, Carbs:24.2 g, Protein:3.8 g, Sugars:4.2 g, Sodium:500 mg

Perky Paleo Potato & Protein Powder _Servings: 1_

Cooking Time: 0 Minutes

Ingredients:

1 small sweet potato, pre-baked and fleshed out 1-Tbsp protein powder

1 small banana, sliced

¼-cup blueberries

¼-cup raspberries

Choice of toppings: cacao nibs, chia seeds, hemp hearts, favorite nut/seed butter (optional)

Directions:

1. In a small serving bowl, mash the sweet potato using a fork. Add the protein powder. Mix well until thoroughly combined.

2. Arrange the banana slices, blueberries, and raspberries on top of the mixture. Garnish with your desired toppings. You can relish this breakfast meal, either cold or warm.

Nutrition Info: Calories 302 Fat: 10g Protein: 15.3g Sodium: 65mg Total Carbs: 46.7g

Tomato Bruschetta With Basil _Servings: 8_

Ingredients:

½ c. chopped basil

2 minced garlic cloves

1 tbsp. balsamic vinegar

2 tbsps. Olive oil

½ tsp. cracked black pepper

1 sliced whole wheat baguette

8 diced ripe Roma tomatoes

1 tsp. sea salt

Directions:

1. First, preheat the oven to 375 F.

2. In a bowl, dice the tomatoes, mix in balsamic vinegar, chopped basil, garlic, salt, pepper, and olive oil, set aside.

3. Slice the baguette into 16-18 slices and for about 10 minutes, place on a baking pan to bake.

4. Serve with warm bread slices and enjoy.

5. For leftovers, store in an airtight container and put in the fridge.

Try putting them over grilled chicken, it is amazing!

<u>Nutrition Info:</u> Calories: 57, Fat:2.5 g, Carbs:7.9 g, Protein:1.4 g, Sugars:0.2 g, Sodium:261 mg

Cinnamon Pancakes With Coconut <u>Servings: 2</u>

Cooking Time: 18 Minutes

Ingredients:

2 organic eggs

1 tbsp almond flour

2oz cream cheese

¼ cup shredded coconut and more for garnishing ½ tbsp erythritol

1/8 tsp salt

1 tsp cinnamon

4 tbsp stevia

½ tbsp olive oil

Directions:

1. Crack eggs in a bowl, beat until fluffy and then beat in flour and cream cheese until smooth.

2. Add remaining ingredients and then stir until well combined.

3. Take a frying pan, place it over medium heat, grease it with oil, then pour in half of the batter and cook for 3 to 4 minutes per side until the pancake has cooked and nicely golden brown.

4. Transfer pancake to a plate and cook another pancake in the same manner by using the remaining batter.

5. Sprinkle coconut on top of cooked pancakes and serve.

<u>Nutrition Info:</u> Calories 575, Total Fat 51g, Total Carbs 3.5g, Protein 19g

Nutty Blueberry Banana Oatmeal <u>*Servings: 6*</u>

Cooking Time: 2 Hours

Ingredients:

2 cup rolled eats

1/4 cup almonds (toasted)

1/4 cup walnuts

1/4 cup pecans

2 tbsp ground flax seeds

1 tsp ground ginger

1 tsp cinnamon

1/4 tsp sea salt

2 tbsp coconut sugar

½ tsp baking powder

2 cups of milk

2 bananas

1 cup fresh blueberries

1 tbsp maple syrup

1 tsp vanilla extract

1 tbsp melted butter

Yogurt for serving

Directions:

1. In a large bowl, add nuts, flax seeds, baking powder, spices, and coconut sugar and mix.

2. In another bowl, beat eggs, milk, maple syrup, and vanilla extract.

3. Slice the bananas in half and layer them in the slow cooker pot with blueberries.

4. Add oats mixture and pour the milk mixture on the top.

5. Drizzle with melted butter,

6. Cook the slow cooker on low heat for 4 hours or on high heat for 4 hours. Cook till the liquid is absorbed and oats are golden brown.

7. Serve warm and top it off with plain Greek yogurt.

Nutrition Info: Calories 346 mg Total Fat: 15g Carbohydrates: 45g Protein: 11g Sugar: 17g Fiber 7g Sodium: 145 mg Cholesterol: 39mg

Poached Salmon Egg Toast _Servings: 2_

Cooking Time: 4 Minutes

Ingredients:

Bread, two slices rye or whole-grain toasted Lemon juice, one quarter teaspoon

Avocado, two tablespoons mashed

Black pepper, one quarter teaspoon

Eggs, two poached

Salmon, smoked, four ounces

Scallions, one tablespoon sliced thin

Salt, one eighth teaspoon

Directions:

1. Add lemon juice to avocado with pepper and salt. Spread the mixed avocado over the toasted bread slices. Lay smoked salmon over toast and top with a poached egg. Top with sliced scallions.

Nutrition Info: Calories 389 fat 17.2 grams protein 33.5 grams carbs 31.5 grams sugar 1.3 grams fiber 9.3 grams

Chia Breakfast Pudding <u>*Servings: 2*</u>

Cooking Time: 0 Minutes

Ingredients:

Chia seeds, four tablespoons

Almond butter, one tablespoon

Coconut milk, three-fourths cup

Cinnamon, one teaspoon

Vanilla, one teaspoon

Cold coffee, three-fourths cup

Directions:

1. Combine all of the fixings well and pour them into a refrigerator-safe container. Cover well and let refrigerate overnight.

<u>Nutrition Info:</u> Calories 282 carbs 5 grams protein 5.9 grams fat 24

grams

Eggs With Cheese _Servings: 1_

Ingredients:

¼ c. chopped tomato

1 egg white

1 chopped green onion

2 tbsps. Fat-free milk

1 slice whole wheat bread

1 egg

½ oz. reduced fat grated cheddar cheese

Directions:

1. Mix the egg and egg whites in a bowl and add the milk.

2. Scramble the mixture in a non-stick frying pan until the eggs cook.

3. Meanwhile, toast the bread.

4. Spoon the scrambled egg mixture onto the toasted bread and top with the cheese until it melts.

5. Add the onion and the tomato.

<u>Nutrition Info:</u> Calories: 251, Fat:11.0 g, Carbs:22.3 g, Protein:16.9

g, Sugars:1.8 g, Sodium:451 mg

Tropical Bowls _Servings: 2_

Cooking Time: 0 Minutes

Ingredients:

1 cup orange juice

1 cup mango, peeled and cubed

1 cup pineapple, peeled and cubed

1 banana, peeled

1 teaspoon chia seeds

A pinch of turmeric powder

4 strawberries, sliced

Directions:

1. In your blender, mix the orange juice with the mango, pineapple, banana, chia seeds and turmeric. Pulse well, divide into bowls, top each with the strawberries and serve.

2. Enjoy!

Nutrition Info: calories 171, fat 3, fiber 6, carbs 8, protein 11

Tex-mex Hash Browns _Servings: 4_

Cooking Time: 30 Minutes

Ingredients:

1 ½ lb. potatoes, sliced into cubes

1 tablespoon olive oil

Pepper to taste

1 onion, chopped

1 red bell pepper, chopped

1 jalapeno, sliced into rings

1 teaspoon oil

½ teaspoon ground cumin

½ teaspoon taco seasoning mix

Directions:

1. Preheat your air fryer to 320 degrees F.

2. Toss potatoes in 1 tablespoon oil.

3. Season with pepper.

4. Transfer to the air fryer basket.

5. Air fry for 20 minutes, shaking twice during cooking.

6. Combine remaining ingredients in a bowl.

7. Add to the air fryer.

8. Mix well.

9. Cook at 356 degrees F for 10 minutes.

Shirataki Pasta With Avocado And Cream

Servings: 2

Cooking Time: 6 Minutes

Ingredients:

½ packet of shirataki noodles, cooked

½ of an avocado

½ tsp cracked black pepper

½ tsp salt

½ tsp dried basil

1/8 cup heavy cream

Directions:

1. Place a medium pot half full with water over medium heat, bring it to boil, then add noodles and cook for 2 minutes.

2. Then drain the noodles and set aside until required.

3. Place avocado in a bowl, mash it with a fork, 4. Mash avocado in a bowl, transfer it in a blender, add remaining ingredients, and pulse until smooth.

5. Take a frying pan, place it over medium heat and when hot, add noodles in it, pour in the avocado mixture, stir well and cook for 2

minutes until hot.

6. Serve straight away.

Nutrition Info: Calories 131, Total Fat 12.6g, Total Carbs 4.9g, Protein 1.2g, Sugar 0.3g, Sodium 588mg

Delicious Amaranth Porridge _Servings: 2_

Cooking Time: 30 Minutes

Ingredients:

½ cup water

1 cup almond milk, unsweetened

½ cup amaranth

1 pear, peeled and cubed

½ teaspoon ground cinnamon

¼ teaspoon fresh ginger, grated

A pinch of ground nutmeg

1 teaspoon maple syrup

2 tablespoons chopped pecans

Directions:

1. Put the water and the almond milk in a pot, bring to a simmer over medium heat, add the amaranth, mix and cook for 20 minutes.

Add the pear, cinnamon, ginger, nutmeg and maple syrup and mix.

Simmer for 10 minutes more, divide into bowls and serve with pecans sprinkled on top.

2. Enjoy!

Nutrition Info: calories 199, fat 9, fiber 4, carbs 25, protein 3

Almond Flour Pancakes With Cream Cheese

Servings: 2

Cooking Time: 18 Minutes

Ingredients:

½ cup almond flour

1 tsp erythritol

½ tsp cinnamon

2oz cream cheese

2 organic eggs

1 tbsp unsalted butter

Directions:

1. Prepare the pancake batter, and for this, place flour in a blender, add remaining ingredients and pulse for 2 minutes until smooth.

2. Tip the batter in a bowl and let it rest for 3 minutes.

3. Then take a large skillet pan, place it over medium heat, add butter and when it melts, pour in ¼ of prepared pancake batter.

4. Spread the batter evenly in the pan, cook for 2 minutes per side until nicely golden brown and then transfer pancake to a plate.

5. Cook three more pancakes in the same manner by using the remaining batter and, when done, serve the pancakes with favorite berries.

Nutrition Info: Calories 170, Total Fat 14.3g, Total Carbs 4.3, Protein 6.9g, Sugar 0.2g, Sodium 81mg

Turkey Apple Breakfast Hash _Servings: 5_

Cooking Time: 10 Minutes

Ingredients:

For the meat:

1 lb. ground turkey

1 tablespoon coconut oil

½ teaspoon dried thyme

½ teaspoon cinnamon

sea salt, to taste

For the hash:

1 tbsp coconut oil

1 onion

1 large apple, peeled, cored, and chopped

2 cups spinach or greens of choice

½ tsp turmeric

½ tsp dried thyme

sea salt, to taste

1 large or 2 small zucchinis

½ cup shredded carrots

2 cups cubed frozen butternut squash (or the sweet potato) 1 tsp cinnamon

¾ tsp powdered ginger

½ tsp garlic powder

Directions:

1. In a skillet, heat a spoonful of coconut oil over medium/high heat.

Attach turkey to the ground and cook until crispy. Season with thyme, cinnamon, and a pinch of sea salt. Move to the plate.

2. Throw remaining coconut oil into the same skillet and sauté onion until softened for 2-3 minutes.

3. Add the courgettes, apple, carrots, and frozen squash to taste—

Cook for around 4-5 minutes, or until veggies soften.

4. Attach and whisk in spinach until wilted.

5. Add cooked turkey, seasoning, salt, and shut off oil.

6. Enjoy this hash fresh from the pan, or let it cool and refrigerate all week long. The hash can remain in a sealed container in the

refrigerator for about 5-6 days.

<u>Nutrition Info:</u> Calories 350 Carbs: 20g Fat: 19g Protein: 28g

Cheesy Flax And Hemp Seeds Muffins _Servings: 2_

Cooking Time: 30 Minutes

Ingredients:

1/8 cup flax seeds meal

¼ cup raw hemp seeds

¼ cup almond meal

Salt, to taste

¼ tsp baking powder

3 organic eggs, beaten

1/8 cup nutritional yeast flakes

¼ cup cottage cheese, low-fat

¼ cup grated parmesan cheese

¼ cup scallion, sliced thinly

1 tbsp olive oil

Directions:

1. Switch on the oven, then set it 360°F and let it preheat.

2. Meanwhile, take two ramekins, grease them with oil, and set aside until required.

3. Take a medium bowl, add flax seeds, hemp seeds, and almond meal, and then stir in salt and baking powder until mixed.

4. Crack eggs in another bowl, add yeast, cottage cheese, and parmesan, stir well until combined, and then stir this mixture into the almond meal mixture until incorporated.

5. Fold in scallions, then distribute the mixture between prepared ramekins and bake for 30 minutes until muffins are firm and the top is nicely golden brown.

6. When done, take out the muffins from the ramekins and let them cool completely on a wire rack.

7. For meal prepping, wrap each muffin with a paper towel and refrigerate for up to thirty-four days.

8. When ready to eat, reheat muffins in the microwave until hot and then serve.

Nutrition Info: Calories 179, Total Fat 10.9g, Total Carbs 6.9g, Protein 15.4g, Sugar 2.3g, Sodium 311mg

Cheesy Cauliflower Waffles With Chives

Servings: 2

Cooking Time: 15 Minutes

Ingredients:

1 cup cauliflower florets

1 tbsp chives, minced

½ tsp cracked black pepper

1 tsp onion powder

1 tsp garlic powder

1 cup shredded mozzarella cheese

½ cup grated parmesan cheese

2 organic eggs, beaten

1 tbsp olive oil

Directions:

1. Switch on the waffle iron, grease it with oil and let it preheat.

2. Meanwhile, prepare the waffle batter and for this, place all its ingredients in a bowl and whisk until combined.

3. Ladle half of the batter into the hot waffle iron, shut it with lid, and cook until nicely golden brown.

4. Take out the waffle and cook another waffle in the same manner by using the remaining batter.

5. For meal prepping, place waffles in an airtight container, separating waffles with a wax paper and store for up to four days.

Nutrition Info: Calories 149, Total Fat 8.5g, Total Carbs 6.1g, Protein 13.3g, Sugar 2.3g, Sodium 228mg

Breakfast Sandwich Servings: 1

Cooking Time: 7 Minutes

Ingredients:

1 frozen breakfast

Directions:

1. Air fry sandwich at 340 degrees F for 7 minutes.

106. Savory Veggie Muffins Servings: 5

Cooking Time: 18-23 Minutes

Ingredients:

¾ cup almond meal

½ tsp baking soda

¼ cup whey Protein concentrate powder

2 teaspoons fresh dill, chopped

Salt, to taste

4 large organic eggs

1½ tablespoons nutritional yeast

2 teaspoons apple cider vinegar

3 tablespoons fresh lemon juice

2 tablespoons coconut oil, melted

1 cup coconut butter, softened

1 bunch scallion, chopped

2 medium carrots, peeled and grated

½ cup fresh parsley, chopped

Directions:

1. Preheat the oven to 350 degrees F. Grease 10 cups of your large muffin tin.

2. In a large bowl, mix together flour, baking soda, Protein powder and salt.

3. In another bowl, add eggs, nutritional yeast, vinegar, lemon juice and oil and beat till well combined.

4. Add coconut butter and beat till mixture becomes smooth.

5. Add egg mixture into flour mixture and mix till well combined.

6. Fold in scallion, carts and parsley.

7. Place the amalgamation into prepared muffin cups evenly.

8. Bake for about 18-23 minutes or till a toothpick inserted inside center comes out clean.

<u>Nutrition Info:</u> Calories: 378, Fat: 13g, Carbohydrates: 32g, Fiber: 11g, Protein: 32g

Zucchini Pancakes _Servings: 8_

Cooking Time: 6-10 Min

Ingredients:

1 cup chickpea flour

1½ cups water, divided

¼ teaspoon cumin seeds

¼ tsp cayenne

¼ teaspoon ground turmeric

Salt, to taste

½ cup zucchini, shredded

½ cup red onion, chopped finely

1 green chile, seeded and chopped finely

¼ cup fresh cilantro, chopped

Directions:

1. In a large bowl, add flour and ¾ cup with the water and beat till smooth.

2. Add remaining water and beat till a thin 3. Fold inside onion, ginger, Serrano pepper and cilantro.

4. Lightly, grease a substantial nonstick skillet with oil and heat on medium-low heat.

5. Add about ¼ cup of mixture and tilt the pan to spread it evenly in the skillet.

6. Cook for around 4-6 minutes.

7. Carefully, alter the side and cook for approximately 2-4 minutes.

8. Repeat while using remaining mixture.

9. Serve together with your desired topping.

Nutrition Info: Calories: 389, Fat: 13g, Carbohydrates: 25g, Fiber: 4g, Protein: 21g

Breakfast Burgers With Avocado Buns *Servings:* 1

Cooking Time: 5 Minutes

Ingredients:

1 ripe avocado

1 egg, pasture-raised

1 red onion slice

1 tomato slice

1 lettuce leaf

Sesame seed for garnish

Salt to taste

Directions:

1. Peel the avocado and remove the seed. Slice the avocado into half. This will serve as the bun. Set aside.

2. Grease a skillet over medium flame and fry the egg's sunny side up for 5 minutes or until set.

3. Assemble the breakfast burger by placing on top of one avocado half with the egg, red onion, tomato, and lettuce leaf.

4. Top with the remaining avocado bun.

5. Garnish with sesame seeds on top and season with salt to taste.

Nutrition Info: Calories 458Total Fat 39gSaturated Fat 4gTotal Carbs 20gNet Carbs 6g,Protein 13gSugar: 8gFiber: 14gSodium: 118mgPotassium 1184mg

Tasty Cheesy And Creamy Spinach Puffs

Servings: 2

Cooking Time: 12 Minutes

Ingredients:

½ cup almond flour

½ tsp garlic powder

½ tsp salt

1 organic egg

1½ tbsp heavy whipping cream

¼ cup feta cheese, crumbled

½ tbsp olive oil

Directions:

1. Switch on the oven, then set its temperature to 350 °F and let it preheat.

2. Meanwhile, prepare the cookie batter, and for this, place all the ingredients in a blender and then pulse for 2 minutes until smooth.

3. Prepare cookies and for this, place prepared batter onto a working space and then shape it with 1-inch balls.

4. Take a cookie sheet, grease it with oil, then arrange cookies on it, with some distance apart, and bake for 12 minutes until cooked and nicely golden.

5. When done, let cookies cool in the cookie sheet for 5 minutes, then transfer them onto a wire rack to cool completely and then serve.

Nutrition Info: Calories 294, Total Fat 24g, Total Carbs 7.8g, Protein 12.2g, Sugar 1.1g, Sodium 840mg

Apple Cinnamon Overnight Oats _Servings: 2_

Ingredients:

1 diced apple

2 tbsps. Chia seeds

½ tbsp. ground cinnamon

½ tsp. pure vanilla extract

1¼ c. nonfat milk

Kosher salt

1 c. old-fashioned rolled oats

2 tsps. Honey

Directions:

1. Divide the oats, chia seeds or ground flaxseed, milk, cinnamon, honey or maple syrup, vanilla extract, and salt into two Mason jars.

Place the lids tightly on top and shake until thoroughly combined.

2. Remove the lids and add half of the diced apple to each jar.

Sprinkle with additional cinnamon, if desired. Place the lids tightly back on the jars and refrigerate for at least 4 hours or overnight.

3. You can store the overnight oats in single-serve containers in the refrigerator for up to 3 days.

Nutrition Info: Calories: 339, Fat:8 g, Carbs:60 g, Protein:13 g, Sugars:15 g, Sodium:161 mg.

Vegetable Egg Hash _Servings: 4_

Cooking Time: 35 Minutes

Ingredients:

Baby new potatoes, quartered – 10 ounces

Zucchini, chopped – 1

Garlic, minced – 2 cloves

Red bell pepper, chopped – 1

Yellow bell pepper, chopped – 1

Green onion, chopped – 2

Extra virgin olive oil – 2 tablespoon

Sea salt – 0.75 teaspoon

Red pepper flakes – 0.5 teaspoon

Eggs, large – 4

Black pepper, ground – 0.25 teaspoon

Directions:

1. Allow your quartered potatoes to boil in a large pot of salted water until fork-tender, about six to eight minutes. Drain them off, discarding the water.

2. Add the quartered baby new potatoes to a large skillet along with the bell peppers, zucchini, garlic, and olive oil. Sprinkle the seasonings for the egg hash over the top and then allow the hash to sauté until the vegetables are browned, about eight to ten minutes.

Be sure to give the hash a good stir every couple of minutes for even cooking.

3. Once the vegetables are ready, use a spoon to create four craters or wells for the eggs to fit into. Crack the eggs into the craters, with one egg per crater. Place a lid on the skillet and allow the eggs to cook until cooked to your preference, about four to five minutes.

4. Remove the skillet of the vegetable egg hash from the heat, sprinkle the green onions over the top, and enjoy the hash and eggs while hot.

Lightning Source UK Ltd.
Milton Keynes UK
UKHW021426310521
384684UK00002B/512